How to Coordinate Services for Students and Families

Larry F. Guthrie

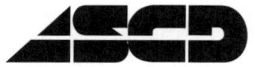

Association for Supervision and Curriculum Development
Alexandria, Virginia

The Author:
Larry F. Guthrie is Director of the Center for Research, Evaluation, and Training in Education (CREATE), 1011 Cabrillo Ave., Burlingame, California 94010; telephone: (415) 579-0880.

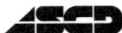

Association for Supervision and Curriculum Development
1250 N. Pitt Street • Alexandria, Virginia 22314
Telephone: (703) 549-9110 • Fax: (703) 299-8631

Gene R. Carter, *Executive Director*
Michelle Terry, *Assistant Executive Director, Program Development*
Ronald S. Brandt, *Assistant Executive Director*
Nancy Modrak, *Managing Editor, ASCD Books*
Stephanie Justen, *Assistant Editor*
Gary Bloom, *Manager, Design and Production Services*
Tracey Smith, *Production Coordinator*
Valerie Sprague, *Desktop Publisher*

Copyright © 1996 by the Association for Supervision and Curriculum Development. All rights reserved. No part of this publication may be reproduced or transmitted in any form or by any means, electronic or mechanical, including photocopy, recording, or any information storage and retrieval system, without permission except as follows: **For current individual ASCD members:** You may make up to 100 copies of one chapter from this book without permission provided that (1) duplication is for one-time academic use in a nonprofit institution and (2) copies are made available without charge to recipients. **For universities:** Requests beyond the above specifications should be submitted to the Copyright Clearance Center, 222 Rosewood Dr., Danvers, MA 01923, USA (phone 508-750-8400, fax 508-750-4470). Copies must cite the source and include an ASCD copyright notice (e.g., copyright 1994 by the Association for Supervision and Curriculum Development). **For school districts:** Contact Mary Riendeau at (703) 549-9110, ext. 404, for permission to make more than 100 copies of any one chapter.

Organizations that wish to reprint rather than photocopy material should contact Mary Riendeau at (703) 549-9110, ext. 404.

ASCD publications present a variety of viewpoints. The views expressed or implied in this book should not be interpreted as official positions of the Association.

Printed in the United States of America.

ASCD Stock No.196001
P2/96

Library of Congress Cataloging-in-Publication Data

Guthrie, Larry F.
   How to coordinate services for students and families / Larry F. Guthrie.
      p. cm.
   Includes bibliographical references.
   ISBN 0-87120-254-9 (pbk.)
    1. School social work—United States. 2. School children-
-Services for—United States—Planning. 3. School children—United States—Social conditions. 4. School health services—United States. I. Association for Supervision and Curriculum Development.
II. Title.
LB3013.4.G88 1996
371.2'022—dc20   95-50170
                                                                                   CIP

99 98 97 96 95   5 4 3 2 1

How to Coordinate Services for Students and Families

1. Introduction   1
2. A Nine-Step Program   17
3. Designing Services   27
4. Staying Alive and Going to Scale   51
References   59

1
Introduction

SEVERAL YEARS AGO, I WAS GIVING AN ALL-DAY WORKSHOP ON improving Chapter 1 services in a rural school district in northern California. I talked about how to incorporate more advanced skills in lessons for students served by Chapter 1 and how to coordinate Chapter 1 lessons with the regular program and curriculum. I led the teachers through several interactive exercises using lots of overheads and handouts. Still, they didn't seem to respond as I'd hoped. At last, one of them spoke up, "All this is interesting, and sure, we need to think about developing higher-order skills. But our kids don't have shoes, and many are coming to school hungry. They need glasses, but can't afford them. Those are our real concerns. What can we do about them?"

The poverty and health concerns confronting those teachers are now common in American schools. Family poverty, community crime, violence, and untreated health needs are part of the fabric of the American classroom. Families are up against more difficult circumstances and are in a much more fragile condition than they were 20 years ago. In many communities, schools are trying to take up the slack with crisis counseling, food and clothing banks, and extra health care—things that in previous generations were taken care of by families, churches, and neighborhoods.

When children come to school hungry, unhealthy, or abused, the responsibility for addressing these needs often falls to teachers and other school personnel by default. They try to do what they can—talking to the child and offering to meet with parents. They may involve the school nurse or counseling staff, but these are also stretched thin and cannot provide direct service. Sometimes, the counselor will refer the student to a local mental health agency or bring in law enforcement. Once this happens, the problem is in someone else's hands and the school is unable to assist in finding a solution.

Schools are in a bind. As educational institutions, their primary focus is on helping students learn and develop as productive, happy citizens. They cannot ignore the personal crises their students are facing, but their resources are limited. They are ill-equipped to meet the needs of all children. They have neither the facilities nor the expertise to do so. Yet, if schools concentrate exclusively on academic improvement, they will almost certainly lose those students most at risk of school failure. Those students will drop out—not only because of poor grades, but for a variety of social and emotional reasons.

School violence and juvenile crime are outgrowths of the same conditions. Here, too, we are looking for alternatives, but there's no clear-cut consensus about what to do. On one side, we hear voices advocating a "get tough" approach. For schools, this translates into tighter discipline and increased school suspension. In the larger community it means "three strikes and you're out," longer prison sentences, and strict limits on welfare (or its elimination). Advocates for the other side dismiss this approach, pointing to mounting evidence that the root causes of these problems are so deeply embedded in society that they will not be affected by quick fixes and stiffer punishments. For example, the head of Florida's department of corrections rejects "prison beds and juvenile boot camps" as possible solutions. In his view, interventions need to be applied much earlier, while young people are still in school (Smolowe 1994).

Increasing numbers of educators, health practitioners, and social service specialists are looking for preventive, longer-term interventions, and a growing number of communities have begun to experiment with how that can work. As they look for points of intervention, they see that what's troubling kids isn't solely poverty, or crime in their community, or the negative influence of drug dealers, or parental neglect, or poor health. It's all of these and more, for troubling conditions seldom come alone. Take Robert, for example.

> Robert is in the 5th grade and lives in public housing with his mother, older sister, and two younger brothers. His mother works part-time, but only makes $6 an hour. She's getting employment training, and receives AFDC and Medicare, but the family can barely make ends meet. Robert's 13-year-old sister, Evelyn, has a medical condition and may need an operation. His father doesn't live with them, but occasionally visits the family on weekends. He seldom helps out with finances. Robert's mother has been looking for day care and after-school care for the younger kids, but has been unsuccessful. Evelyn takes care of the boys in the evening while their mother works. Last year, in the 4th grade, Robert was a fairly good student, but now his grades have dropped and he's become disruptive in class. On several occasions, his teacher sent him to the principal, who finally contacted Robert's mother. His mother expressed concern, but said she didn't know what to do; Robert had recently started hanging out with a group of older kids. She said she's reaching the end of her rope with him and everything else.

The system is not neglecting Robert and his family. His mother receives food stamps and AFDC. They live in public housing. Robert is in a Chapter 1 class at school, and his sister's medical treatment is subsidized. Unfortunately, none of these programs appears to be making much of a difference. The family is still poor, Robert's grades are not improving, and his sister is still sick. What they need is some assistance that takes their overall situation into consideration and coordinates the help they're getting. The school needs to know what's going on in the other parts of Robert's life, and so do the other agencies and providers.

Our Non-System

Schools do not operate in isolation to help solve these problems. In fact, a vast array of government and private agencies, and community-based organizations serve at-risk children and youth, and their families. County welfare agencies, child protection agencies, juvenile courts, youth employment programs, health and mental health programs, child care programs, and early childhood development agencies are all offering assistance to needy children and youth. At the federal level, there are more than 170 programs for children and youth (GAO). At the state level, it's the same story. California services for children, for instance, are distributed through more than 160 programs in 35 agencies and seven departments (Kirst and McLaughlin 1989). This is only the government; scores of private counseling, day care, and other institutions add to the mix.

With all these agencies and programs, you'd expect our children to be better off than they are, but there's nothing that ties the programs together. An estimated $300 billion is spent on children's services in this country and still they make up the poorest segment of the society. Services are overlapping and disconnected, and agencies are compartmentalized (Hodgkinson 1989, Schorr 1988). They are part of an elaborate bureaucracy where the left hand doesn't know what the right one is doing.

It has been estimated that a low-income family in an urban community would have to apply to 18 different agencies to get the kind of assistance its members might be eligible for (Osborne and Gaebler 1993). If we had to buy our groceries that way, each aisle in your local Safeway would be in another part of the city, far from where most people live. To get milk you'd have to go here; fruits and vegetables would be across town (Kirst 1992). That's no way to run a supermarket, and it's no way to provide assistance to needy children and families.

What's Not Working

We got into this fix because the system is based on *programs*. Education, health, social services—in fact, all of our government services—are based on a system of programs that contribute to the unwieldy tangle of services we have today. Instead of a set of inter-locking and complementary services, the national emphasis on specialization has created a jumble of single-issue programs. The current system meets one need at a time. A new program is designed to put out each new fire. Each symptom has its own "cure." Students drop out, so we institute a dropout prevention program. Low grades are met with a special remedial class; poor nutrition gets a lunch program; and low-income mothers are given AFDC support.

The programs are not inherently bad. Individually, each targets a critical problem and offers services to clients who need them. What is wrong is the way the existing system is set up. It is fundamentally at odds with how the needs of children and families occur—and how they should be met. Needs like those of Robert's family don't come neatly separated and packaged; they are intertwined and connected. Providing help in one area, such as Robert's disruptive behavior in class, is unlikely to affect his other, more critical concerns. Here are some examples of what's not working in our current set-up of programs:

1. Interventions are short-term. Few agencies, including schools, are able to take a protracted, developmental perspective in designing and providing assistance. Mental-health counseling, for example, may be two weeks, while academic assistance may last a semester. We all hear of the welfare mothers who make a career of staying on public assistance, but the programs designed to get them off welfare are often limited in scope. The predicaments families find themselves in don't just appear overnight; they develop and ferment for years and may take years to improve.

2. Getting to services is a challenge. Finding where services are offered and getting there are the first hurdles. Then, the application and review process for eligibility is a confusing maze of offices, forms, and rules. The poorest and most troubled families, many of whom may not be fluent in English, are those least able to navigate their way through the bureaucracy. As a result, their needs often go unmet causing whatever hopes for school success the children might have to go out the window.

Within each program, the kinds of services and who gets them are determined by sets of complex rules and regulations. School personnel are all too familiar with the testing, paperwork, and reporting requirements that accompany categorical and other special funding. Just as standardized tests and other assessments slot children into particular programs in schools, each agency houses a variety of programs with its own set of assessments and eligibility requirements. Very often, eligibility is based on income, family structure, or some other deficit criterion.

Some communities, especially those in rural areas, simply don't have every form of assistance available. If they do, the hours of operation or location may be a problem (McCart 1993). People who have jobs, for example, find it hard to go in the middle of the day. Others don't have cars and can't drive across town. We also know that there are barriers to access in the offices themselves: endless, duplicative paperwork and impersonal, officious clerks who make seeking help a humiliating experience.

3. People in schools and other agencies don't work together. Administrators and staff in one agency seldom know much about how other agencies are organized and operate. For example, how familiar are school administrators with the social service agencies in the community? Ask yourself how much you know about what social workers or public health professionals do. The school principal may routinely refer students to one agency or another, or contact them when a particular need arises, yet, the relationships are formal and crisis-driven. On occasions when the school contacts other agencies, very often the child or family may have to go to several because the initial referral was incorrect. Teachers have even less contact with the service personnel in other agencies, despite the fact they are all trying to help the same child and family.

4. Programs protect their turf. Once a program is funded and operational, a lot of effort goes into continuing the funding and maintaining staff positions. Money, staff, and status become tied up in the program, and any change in the system represents a potential threat to the program and its administrators. This doesn't mean the programs are doing a poor job, but the emphasis on self-preservation and maintaining the status quo makes them resistant to change and cooperation (Hodgkinson 1989).

5. The system isn't concerned about self-improvement. In our system, what's typically evaluated is the *process*, not the *product*. We measure the number and type of services provided and kids served, rather than the results of those services. The numbers are used to promote the program, not to manage it. As long as a dropout prevention program provides counseling to 25 potential dropouts per month, then the program director is satisfied and so is the funder. Do they ever ask how many children actually stay in school? How many of them graduate? These questions are harder to answer because it takes time and effort to track the results. Nevertheless, these are the only questions that *really* matter.

6. Programs don't view clients as customers. In most government programs, the people served are treated only as numbers. With huge caseloads and strict procedures, workers assume they have to take a dispassionate position. Even the terminology—"cases," not "families"—is deliberately impersonal. Instead of tailoring services to address the particular troubles of families, programs take a one-size-fits-all approach. Everyone who qualifies gets the same thing.

What Might Work

Despite this bleak picture, there is reason for hope. Critics of the present system are being heard in caucus rooms and board rooms where federal and state policies are shaped. The federal government and some states are passing legislation that encourages cooperation and attempts to break down barriers and cut red tape. In addition, parts of the system are beginning to work together. The benefit of integrating services and building coalitions among agencies has started to make sense to policymakers, administrators, and service providers across the various service sectors. Agency leaders are talking to each other, and several communities have established procedures for periodic networking and information-sharing.

At the federal level, legislation such as the Family Support Act of 1988, the Job Training Partnership Act, and Even Start under Title 1 require states to develop interagency councils to coordinate planning and service delivery as a condition for federal funds (McCart 1993). Even Start focuses on improving adult literacy and children's school readiness through cooperative arrangements that bring pre-schools and adult education programs together.

Vice President Albert Gore's National Performance Review on reinventing government has recommended consolidating funds for more than 50 categorical programs as well as using block grants to allow state and local governments more discretion in how money from federal grants is distributed (Gore 1993).

Change is underway at the state level, too. In California, Healthy Start is directed at developing school-linked services in communities. Funded by the state legislature in 1991, the program provides funding to local communities for integrating services. The program targets children most in need—those on welfare or limited-English proficient—and can include a range of services from health care, immunizations, and family counseling to drug abuse and prevention. Specific design of the collaboration may vary from one community to the next.

In Kentucky, Family Resource Centers and Youth Services Centers are set up in or near schools where one-fifth or more of the students are eligible for free and reduced lunch. The Family Resource Centers provide a set of core services at elementary schools including preschool and after-school day care, prenatal education, parent and child education, training for day-care providers, and health services. The Youth Services Centers are for schools with students over the age of 12. They provide referrals for health and social services, employment services, summer and part-time job development, drug and alcohol abuse counseling, family crisis and mental health counseling, and more (Russo and Lindle 1994).

The way funding is made available to local communities is also changing. Tennessee, for example, has allowed state service agencies to share costs of services they would otherwise provide separately. Under new policies, child welfare, mental health, and juvenile justice agencies jointly support family preservation services (McCart 1993). Iowa has pooled several funding sources to give pilot counties discretion in allocating money, and Maryland lets communities shift money ear-marked for foster care into preventive services, such as intensive counseling. Block grants are another way states give local entities more flexibility in spending dollars.

In turn, local communities have begun to reorganize themselves in order to provide less fragmented services. San Diego's New Beginnings, for example, formed a cadre of workers from different agencies to work as case managers at a school site and renamed them Family Service Advocates. Health services are provided by the nurse practitioners. Collaboration is supported through a management team of decision makers from participating agencies (Payzant 1992).

Most of these developments are in their infancy. Many are pilot efforts and because of that we don't know if they're going to succeed—or even be around five years from now. While that's true, there also seems to be a clear and growing dissatisfaction with the status quo. Each of these initiatives, whether at a national, state, or local level, is looking for ways to distribute and coordinate the activities of various agencies so that children's services are improved.

Schools and communities need to look at the social and emotional needs of children and families and pinpoint ones the school is best suited to handle, which can best be provided by other institutions and agencies, and which can best be accomplished by joint efforts. The challenge is not simply to divide up responsibilities, but to reconceptualize the role of the school and the relationship between the school, social service agencies, the community, and the larger society. The new arrangement needs to shift the emphasis of each agency away from itself and its traditional function, and toward children and their families. In other words, we need to create a customer-driven, rather than program-driven system of services.

What about the cost? To a large extent, pioneer efforts at interagency collaboration have relied on an infusion of new funds to jump-start activities and build regular communication and coordination across agencies and services. Most pilot efforts have been the result of foundation or special grant support during start-up, not because someone found a way to redistribute money that was already in the community (Gardner 1994).

A wide variety of government and foundation grants are available to support new efforts. Given increasingly tight federal, state, county, and local budgets, however, it's probably a mistake to count on additional funding, even for start-up. It seems clear that competition for scarce resources will only get worse in coming years. Not everyone can be a pilot or demonstration site, and where funds will come after the pilot phase will remain a question. Until there are fundamental changes in how government funds education and social programs, communities interested in collaboration will need to think seriously about creative financing. There are hopeful signs in that direction—in the kinds of discussions now going on in statehouses, county governments, and in local schools and service agencies. But we shouldn't wait for national reforms that may take years to set in motion and even longer to reach the local level. Schools and communities need to think about what they can do now. That's the focus of this book: what you can do *now* to improve conditions for children and families.

Some Basic Ingredients of Interagency Collaboration

The idea that better ways must be found for providing children's services is gaining acceptance around the country. Social service personnel, legislators, and educators are coming to realize that the current set of compartmentalized programs are an insult to our children. Vice President Gore's commission on Reinventing Government concerned this issue in part (Gore 1993). Communities are beginning to find ways to encourage collaboration among agencies and better integrate services. Pilot collaborative projects, interagency networks, conferences, and new legislation also reflect this trend.

As these pioneer efforts unfold, every community can begin to initiate its own collaborative experiment. Just as all politics are local, improved services for children will develop in the contexts of particular communities, schools, and service agencies. There are, of course, no easy answers—no canned programs to insert and no formulas for what works best in one place or another. The strategy for coordination that brings services together in one community might not work in the next. The set of agencies involved and the ways in which schools connect with social services, health, or community-based organizations will differ from community to community. Even without proven models of collaboration, recent experience gives us some clues about how to proceed. We aren't starting empty-handed.

Interagency collaboration can be approached in a variety of ways and at different levels. At the service level, for example, professional coordinators (or case managers) can be assigned to a school to coordinate the services of several agencies and match them with the needs of children and their families. Another scenario might place various agencies at the school, providing easy access and close coordination. At the management or administrative level, cross-agency committees can develop consistent communication and joint projects that allow all educational, mental health, correctional, and other institutions to work with each other. Whatever approach is taken, the overriding purpose should be to meet the needs of children and families. This means that the services should be both *effective* and *user friendly*.

Effective Services

Effective services meet the current needs of clients and prevent more critical problems from developing. Work in interagency collaboration suggests that effective services are comprehensive and preventive. To maintain their effectiveness, they include professional development opportunities for staff and use evaluations to improve the way services are delivered.

To be comprehensive, the set of agencies involved should, as a group, provide a wide spectrum of essential services and attempt to meet the most important needs of those most at risk. Rather than concentrate on the single-issue approach that dominates city and county services, involved agencies should seek ways to ensure that individual children and families receive a *coherent* program of assistance. Often, schools and agencies serve the same children and families but don't realize it. Each agency or program needs to take into account what the partner agencies do and how they fit into an overall matrix.

Implementation will not be easy. Long-standing habits and bureaucratic barriers must fall. Communities must learn about different agencies—how they operate and how to best connect with them. From an agency's point of view there may be no tangible incentive to collaboration; in fact, it probably will mean giving up something. To be successful, each party will have to surrender some turf. As potential funders come to recognize the power of collaboration, additional funding may actually be tied to whether agencies can and do work together.

In preventive services, the needs of children and families are more important than institutional concerns. Under the current system, services do not begin until children are in critical condition. For example, mental health services are offered only to the most emotionally disturbed. Academically, students have to be failing before they are eligible for special help. By the time they get into a program, students are so far behind that their confidence is shot and they've long since given up.

Instead, the system needs to focus on prevention and on how to accommodate students with different backgrounds, cultures, and ways of learning. It should be able to monitor the progress and development of all children, providing special assistance when needed. In practice, this will probably mean a major change in the regular school program. It may also mean that some person (a teacher, social worker, or counselor) will need to take primary responsibility for each child. Student study teams, discussed later, might be one way to make this work.

Another approach could be to shift resources from acute intervention programs into preventive approaches such as prenatal care, health care, day care, and preschool. These may not make a big difference right away, but as the Committee for Economic Development (1985) points out, putting resources into children is an investment not a cost. McCart (1993) summarizes research of the federal government suggesting that each dollar invested in childhood immunizations can reap a savings of $10 in later medical costs.

Interagency collaboration demands that everyone involved develop new ways to serve children and families. They will need time to work out how best to do this. As people develop new skills and learn how to do a new thing better, their commitment to the enterprise increases. This in turn produces better outcomes for clients (Louis and Miles 1990). It's important that professional development and learning be integral to the on-going interagency effort. If you invest only in an occasional workshop on a special topic, you won't see many results. On-site staff will need to communicate regularly and network with others involved in collaborative initiatives.

As interagency collaboration develops, staff will learn to work in new ways that encourage cooperation across agencies. Those involved at all levels will need to acquire new process skills such as coordination, team building, and working together. Staff will learn how to carry out the specialized tasks associated with child and family needs assessment, service plan development, and case management and review. They should be cross-trained to learn about each others' home agency and how it functions. In this way, repositioned staff will develop a more balanced and comprehensive view of the situations of children and their families and the kinds of treatments that might be available.

Collaboration is judged on the impact it has on kids and families—not simply on the steps followed. It's still too early to know how effective the current experiments will be, but as they develop, and we monitor their progress, we must look at *what they accomplish*, not just *what they do*. Streamlined procedures, school-based services, and a better working relationship among agencies are means, not ends, in themselves. All too often, programs are rewarded for merely going through the paces of what they said they would do rather than making a difference for those they're supposed to be helping.

User-friendly Services

Making services user friendly doesn't mean that assistance is provided on a silver platter. It does mean that prospective recipients don't have to waste their time and that of the providers in unnecessary travel, screening, and bureaucratic rigmarole. Help should be accessible, child- and family-centered, and flexible. Services should be within reach in terms of location, hours of operation, and paperwork. They might be co-located at the school, community center, or public housing complex to provide "one-stop shopping." When families need clothes and food, some schools form a food bank or clothes closet. Hours of operation are extended or adjusted to accommodate those who cannot come during the day. Eligibility criteria are streamlined so that parents don't have to go through the same steps over and over again. Agencies might also arrange for staff to devote more than the usual amount of time to the children and families they serve, working early or late or on weekends to match the times when working parents are free.

One of the challenges in many communities is simply getting parents to come to the school so they can learn about available assistance. Some schools provide transportation when families don't have cars. Other schools have set up a parents' room with washing machines and educational materials parents can borrow to use with their children. These approaches help the parents view the school as open and welcoming.

When services are child- and family-centered, agencies cooperate to develop the best, most appropriate response to the pressing needs of children and their families. They take a balanced, comprehensive, long-term view of what will really make a difference and measure success in terms of the child's or family's condition, not on how many services are delivered. In addition, someone on the service end takes responsibility for checking and monitoring the overall situation of the child and family. Some have called this a customer-driven approach.

Traditional "projects" slice the child and family any number of ways without taking a long-term view. A focus on the customer means sharing information, and reducing the competition across agencies, especially between school staff and those from social services and other agencies. As Heath and McLaughlin assert, school staff are "notoriously unaware of services available through juvenile justice, social service, or mental health agencies" (1989, p. 309). Even if they suspect a child's school failure is related to problems at home, teachers typically don't know where to turn for help.

To move from program-driven to child-centered services, we also need to improve our understanding of children's needs and strengths, monitor them over time, and take a broader, more contextual view of how to help. To do this, we need to improve ways of collecting, maintaining, and sharing information on children and families. In some agencies, staff don't even know how many kids are receiving what kinds of service. Child and family services also need to respond to the growing diversity in our communities— diversity not only of ethnicity, language, and culture, but also of needs (Kirst and McLaughlin 1989). Drugs, crime, AIDS, and poverty have become so prevalent that our schools are facing challenges very different from those of 10 —or even five—years ago.

An improved system needs flexibility in its relations with clients and in the way staff respond to clients' needs. At present, the services children receive are often predetermined by rigid sets of procedures and regulations; screening, referral, and the type and length of treatment are all prescribed from the beginning. Children who are eligible for X Program, receive Y Service, no matter what. As we have seen, though, problems don't come in neat packages and treating them through rigid adherence to guidelines results in fragmented, overlapping services. In addition, the way kids are identified and treated can have long-lasting effects on the types of services they receive and, on who they ultimately become. Once children are pigeonholed into a category (dropout, drug abuser, pregnant teen), their fate within the system is often sealed.

Agency staff roles should also be more flexible. At times, service providers may need to step outside the boundaries of their job descriptions to make sure that what needs doing gets done. For example, Schorr (1988) suggests several ways that service can be continued when staff and clients develop close relationships. Staff may step outside their office to provide services in the home or after hours, or use their own car to make sure a parent or child gets to an appointment. In other words, they persevere, doing whatever they must to reach those who need the help most. In a flexible system, rules are bent if they do not work for families. Currently, in many programs, staff are arbitrarily assigned to clients. Perhaps a better way would be to link staff with families of similar cultural background, or because they are familiar with other members of the family. If the current method of assigning staff isn't working, we should be able to make whatever adjustments are necessary to provide the best assistance.

In summary, coordinated services must be both effective and user friendly.

Effective Services:

Comprehensive: making a variety of essential services available to children and families.

Preventive: heading off crises by intervening early and with support.

Training-focused: training staff to work in new ways that encourage cooperation across agencies.

Results-based: collaboration is judged by the impact it has on kids and families, not simply on the steps followed and services delivered.

User-Friendly Services:

Accessible: not burdened with extensive paperwork and located within reach of families and their children.

Child and Family-Centered: the needs of children and families are more important than institutional concerns.

Flexible: rules can be bent.

2
A Nine-Step Program

IN THIS CHAPTER, I OFFER A NINE-STEP PROGRAM FOR BUILDING interagency collaboration (see also Guthrie and Guthrie 1991, Melaville and Blank 1991, Melaville and Blank 1993). The nine steps (Figure 2.1) I outline are by no means comprehensive or complete; they are meant to be general guideposts. If you'd like to supplement or compare them, check out one of the other documents cited above.

FIGURE 2.1
A Nine-Step Program

Step 1: Map the Territory	What programs do the school and other agencies currently offer?
Step 2: Survey the Field	What are school-linked services all about and what's going on in my community or nearby?
Step 3: Review Current Needs and Services	What are the basic needs of families and children in my community? Are there gaps or overlaps in service? Problems of access?
Step 4: Agree on a Common Vision	What do we hope the collaboration will look like in five years?
Step 5: Set Goals and Expectations	What do we want to achieve in terms of children's education and health, the family's security, and relationships among service agencies?
Step 6: Design Comprehensive Services	Which services will be offered, for whom, and where?
Step 7: Develop a Plan	What are the steps to take and when will we take them?
Step 8: Arrange for an Evaluation	How will we know if it's working and how to make it work better?
Step 9: Get to Work	What are we waiting for?

17

Step 1: Map the Territory

The first step toward building a collaboration is to find out who your potential (and probable) partners might be. Make an inventory of all the agencies that currently interact with the school and list the services provided, number of clients, basic eligibility criteria, and the name and number of a contact person for each. An example of a service matrix is provided in Figure 2.2. Start by listing this information for programs administered by the schools, such as Free and Reduced Lunch, Chapter 1, or parenting teens programs. This is your own first cut at a tool your collaborative will later use to assess the quality of current services. Don't think too much about the future uses of the matrix. For now, just concentrate on finding out who the players are and don't worry so much about who's doing a good job or what's missing. As you fill in the information, don't mistake the map for the territory; the picture of social services you have now might not accurately reflect what's really there.

FIGURE 2.2

Sample Services Matrix

Agency or program name	Services provided	Clients: eligibility criteria and number	Contact person	Name, address, and phone number
Title 1	Before and after school tutoring	CTBS scores and teacher recommendation / 40	Title 1 Resource Teacher	School / 583-0900
Free and Reduced Lunch				
Agency 1				
Agency 2				
Agency 3				

Next, try to identify other agencies in the community that are currently involved with the school. The local departments of social services, health, and mental health are an obvious place to begin. Find out, in general terms, how they are connected with families in your school. Next, look for the private agencies, nonprofits, and community-based organizations involved with the school. These may be offering a tutoring program or providing counseling to troubled families. Finally, try to locate other agencies that aren't directly working with the schools. Check with city and county governments for leads and be sure to include private programs. You might even check the Yellow Pages; clinics and other community-based organizations will often be listed there.

As a final step in mapping the territory, you'll need to figure out who you can count on, from the other schools and agencies, to be the main players in a collaboration effort. Who can work with you and assume some of the responsibilities connected with developing the plan and getting it underway? Who can you rely on to stay with it? Find these people and get them on board. The sooner you involve them in the collaborative enterprise, the better. But don't be surprised if they don't all follow through. Integrating services is hard work. It involves a shift in how things are done and threatens the security of people and agencies. Not everyone you approach will want to get involved.

Step 2: Survey the Field

The information provided in this book only scratches the surface of existing models and strategies for interagency collaboration. Before putting together your own collaboration, find out what others are doing to improve interagency collaboration. Consult some of the references listed here or check with your library or university. There are some excellent resources available to help you think about and initiate a school-linked services effort. Many give capsule descriptions of collaborations in various parts of the country (see Bruner 1991, Melaville and Blank 1991, or Melaville and Blank 1993).

Next, follow up on your own leads. You've probably heard of a community or school nearby that has begun to explore alternatives for coordinating children's services. Meet with them and find out what they're doing. Try to identify the strengths of the community as well, such as churches, service organizations, clubs, or neighborhood community centers. Start with the government agencies and community-based organizations. Are any of them working together? In what ways? Are they thinking about strengthening their ties? Contact them to find out what they've done and whether they have any descriptive materials to share (vision statements, proposals, strategies, plans, brochures) that will give you a better idea of what they are doing. Pick their brains. If it sounds as if they're having some success, arrange a visit—not for the purpose of adopting their program, but to build up your own repertoire of ideas, approaches, and options.

If you're the interagency pioneer in your area and aren't aware of other efforts nearby, try to find a state or regional network that can point you in the right direction. County agencies or other intermediate service agencies are a good place to start. You might also try the local department of social services. In addition, you could contact some of the resources listed in various publications about school-linked services. The main idea in this phase is simply to learn as much about improving school-linked services as you can. Do your homework.

Step 3: Review Current Needs and Services

Once you have an idea of who the players are, assess the current needs of children and families in your community as well as available services. In doing this, it will be helpful to ask yourself some questions: What led you to be concerned with the kinds of services children and their families are receiving? What are the most critical needs of children? Are they being met? Is there an agreed-upon set of criteria for who's "at risk?"

While individual programs may be available for students having a wide variety of needs, the formal identification, diagnosis, and referral system may focus on only a few indicators. Look for gaps, redundancies, and weaknesses in services. Don't just rely on what planning-committee members know—look carefully at the data schools and agencies have collected. Then, to complete the picture, interview or survey administrators, community members, teachers, parents, and students.

You might want to start with a statistical picture of the community. Bruner, Bell, Brindis, Chang, and Scarbrough (1993) outline several ways to gather baseline information. Start with community demographics (income levels, employment, and housing) available from the U.S. Bureau of the Census. Next, you might get public health data such as immunization and disease rates. Check with your local health department. Education data should cover things such as student enrollment (with breakdowns by ethnicity and English proficiency), Chapter 1, special education, free or reduced-price lunch eligibility, student achievement, school completion, attendance, and per-pupil expenditures. The school district or state education agency should have this information. Finally, your collaboration might be interested in juvenile crime and incarceration data. Bruner and others suggest contacting the police department and other juvenile justice agencies. Some of this information may already have been compiled in the Annie E. Casey Foundation's *Kids Count Data Book*, issued annually.

Once you have a handle on community demographics, assess the strengths and weaknesses of your potential partner agencies and estimate the level of coordination among programs and services. How do they fit into the system as a whole? Are there gaps in service, overlaps, or problems of access? Is there a case management system that gives an overview of the number and types of services individual students are receiving?

A way to review agencies and their services coordination is to expand upon the matrix you put together in Step 1. The point of entry into the new matrix should be *needs*, rather than *agency* or *program*. List the needs you've identified in your school or community. You might look for academic assistance, personal counseling, substance abuse counseling, employment, and health services. Now match them with the various service providers. This activity should help reveal gaps in service and areas of overlap. Potential roadblocks to coordination (such as regulations or budget requirements) might surface as well.

Step 4: Agree on a Common Vision

Try to capture your team's shared vision of interagency collaboration. Think about how you would like to see children's services provided. What would the program look like? How would agencies and their representatives interact? How would children be identified and served? You might start with the principles outlined in Chapter 1. Are these part of your vision? How could services be made effective and user-friendly? How could you make services more comprehensive, preventive, results-based, accessible, child- and family-centered, and flexible? Bear in mind that other agencies may bring different perspectives and concerns. Make sure you include partners from a variety of backgrounds and with different perspectives (Melaville and Blank 1993). Your vision is not just a written statement you pull out when visitors come; it is a reflection of the values that guide your daily activities.

The collaboration's vision should be clarified early to avoid problems with communication later on. Write it down and agree on the wording. As you begin to develop the collaboration, you will want to return to the vision to ensure that you're on track. A clear vision statement is a good way to keep everyone focused on what is best for children—not the organizations and individuals involved. This doesn't mean the vision should be static. Over time, your vision may evolve into something quite different as you and your partners learn from each other and develop new ideas about what is possible (Senge 1990).

Vision statements don't have to be lengthy or elaborate; in fact, as Louis and Miles (1990) demonstrate, they can be expressed like a motto or slogan. One high school they studied had as its vision: "a school for students and a university for teachers" (p. 219). They mention as well the vision common to many inner-city schools: a place "where all children can learn" (p. 219). Melaville and Blank (1993) quote the vision of the Youth Futures Authority in Savannah-Chatham County, Georgia: "Every child will grow up healthy, be secure, and become literate and economically productive" (p. 44).

Developing a shared vision isn't as easy as it sounds and the process isn't well understood (Fullan 1992). Louis and Miles (1990) caution that a "blueprinted" vision isn't likely to work, and they stress that developing the vision is a joint process and must involve give-and-take among the players. Stay open to different views and don't let some people retreat into passive observation (Fullan 1992). Louis and Miles (1990) suggest that a "back to the future" approach might help some people to think more divergently (p. 293). You might ask your group, for example, to respond to the following: "It's the year 2000. The local newspaper has just written an extensive piece on the community's collaboration among schools and other agencies. What does the headline say?"

Step 5: Set Goals and Expectations

Your goals and expectations should help you to put your vision into action. First, pull out the needs assessment for children and youth in the community and review the matrix of needs and services. Next, try to predict what outcomes you can reasonably expect for children and their families. What would you hope to see, for example, in the areas of education, health, and family security? What changes do you foresee in how agencies work and how would you like interactions among them to be? As you work through the planning phase, you will probably want to modify and refine your expectations. Throughout, the primary focus should be on the partner agencies and how they can work together to improve the services for children and youth. Keep in mind, however, that each organization will have its own set of needs and priorities. They will be coming to the collaboration having tried to accomplish certain goals for years, even decades, and a shift in focus might not come easily.

Some important goals will reach beyond the agencies involved. For example, the team might want to explore ways to tap both public and private resources. In this case, someone will need to assume the task of monitoring new legislation. Exerting influence on policymakers for future funding might be another goal. For this, you might want to share lessons learned from the collaborative process.

Step 6: Design Comprehensive Services

A critical part of the plan will be coming up with the right set of services to meet your needs. Many of these will already be in place—some may need to be enhanced or upgraded, others will have to be created from scratch. Pull out the matrix again. Using the other background information you've gathered, begin to design a set of services that is not only comprehensive, but preventive, flexible, and child-centered. The next chapter goes into detail about some of the key design questions you'll face in creating a school-linked services effort, but a few general points can be made here.

First, make sure you clarify the role that each agency and its representatives will play in the collaborative process. This applies not only to the planning and development stage, but also to the actual integration of services. In planning, try to share assignments fairly; don't let one person shoulder all the responsibility. Build a spirit of collaboration from the beginning. In addition, watch out for the "NIH syndrome," which stands for "Not Invented Here" (Kanter 1992). Organizations often resist importing ideas they didn't come up with themselves. Every institution has its own set of rules and regulations, as well as its own culture made up of values, rites, rituals, and heroes (Deal and Kennedy 1982). Along the way, you'll need to share some of these, because each agency operates under certain constraints that will affect its participation in the collaboration. Mental health service agencies, for example, are restricted by law from disclosing information about their clients, even though information about parents of at-risk children may be crucial for other agencies as they develop a program for the child. Keep in mind that the heavy caseloads of some agencies may have forced them to focus only on the most serious cases. A shift toward prevention may be difficult for them to sell within their organization.

Step 7: Develop a Plan

A project is only as good as the plan it's based on. No matter how urgent the need to collaborate, taking time for careful planning will pay off in the long run. Pull together a core team of people you believe will devote the time and energy necessary to develop a plan and put it into action. The plan should include how you intend to go from thinking to action. Once you've got a planning team together that includes representatives from key agencies, start to sketch out the elements of a plan.

Next, chart the action steps. Formulate what the planning committee or task force will do to improve interagency collaboration. It's a good idea to develop a flowchart or timeline that shows what will be done, who will do it, and when it will be complete. Make sure the flowchart is jointly developed and agreed upon by all involved agencies. Later, the chart can serve as a guide and a check to make sure each agency is holding up its end, and events are on schedule. You might want to include how you will ensure information sharing and day-to-day communication.

Step 8: Arrange for an Evaluation

In these times of belt-tightening budgets, accountability takes on added importance. Unfortunately, many people don't think of evaluating their program until after it is well under way and it's too late to gather the necessary data. A good evaluation requires careful planning, and a good place to start is the *Evaluators' Handbook* (Herman, Morris, and Fitz-Gibbon 1987). Whether you conduct the evaluation yourself or get outside assistance, make sure you're asking both summative (outcome) and formative (project improvement) questions. To get useful answers, you'll need to go beyond counting the number of children served or adding up contact hours. Ask instead: How effective was the collaborative? Has communication improved? Have some of the bureaucratic barriers fallen? Are services for children more effective and timely? How can interagency collaboration be further improved? What will increase efficiency and effectiveness?

Decide beforehand what data you'll need to answer your outcomes question and how you will collect it; otherwise, data collection will be difficult and time-consuming after the fact.

Step 9: Get to Work

The first rule for getting to work is to start small. Don't expect to have everyone involved in joint projects right away. You are dealing with entrenched habits and practices, so begin with clearly manageable tasks. Schedule monthly or biweekly meetings. As you cover the first two phases (map the territory and survey the field) the agencies involved will learn about each other and establish ties. As you reach the planning phase, think in terms of pilot projects rather than massive change efforts.

The final rule of getting to work is to do just that. Fullan (1992) stresses that you shouldn't squander precious staff time in the beginning on needs assessment and program design; these issues will become clearer through *practice*. Carving out visions and planning how things are going to be are seductive activities, but they are also activities that carry little risk. Sooner or later you will need to join your collective hands and throw open the doors.

3
Designing Services

ONCE YOU IDENTIFY YOUR POTENTIAL PARTNERS AND THE RECIPIENTS of improved services, the next step is to figure out who will offer what services for whom and where they will be available. In other words, you need to create a design for your interagency collaborative. This chapter discusses several design features you and others on your team should consider. It also raises some red flags to look out for as you begin to put your plan in motion.

Keep in mind that this is *your* collaboration; you know your situation better than anyone else. How you create the collaboration should depend more on what you and your partners think will work than on well-known or existing models, or what experts say. No strict formula or blueprint for designing school-linked services exists, but there are strategies and approaches that have worked for others and might work for you. In the last few years, we have learned a lot about what might work better and what to avoid.

Perhaps the most important thing at this point is to stick to your vision of what you'd like the collaboration to accomplish. As you start working together, it's easy to fall back on more traditional, familiar approaches that won't have an impact on children and families. When you decide what the collaboration will look like, be conscious of the potential threats to ego, control, and power that can emerge. Be sensitive to what representatives of your own and other agencies might feel as you steer toward a shared vision of more integrated services. Some collaborations find it useful—when power, control, or turf start to become issues—to remind themselves of their overriding purpose and to keep focused on the children and their families.

School personnel often get the mistaken idea that collaboration means adding new programs and services—and more work. In some instances, that's been true. Ideally, however, collaboration will mean that the school is not so much adding on services as forming alliances with existing services and developing new ones from what both camps have already been doing.

If you're working within the constraints of a state initiative or other funding opportunity, it should be easy to see how the suggestions in this chapter fit into the framework you have been provided. Additional guidance can be found in Melaville and Blank's *Together We Can* (1993) or *What It Takes* (1991). Both are excellent resources.

FIGURE 3.1
Design Decisions

Leadership	Who's in charge?
Location of services	Where will services be offered?
Types of services	What services will be provided?
Staffing	Who will provide services?
Targeting	What clients will receive which services?
Cost and budgeting	How will you pay for the collaboration?
Evaluation	How will you know what's working?

FIGURE 3.2
Pitfalls to Avoid

Governance	Creating a new bureaucracy.
Location of services	Putting collaborative services only at the school.
Service delivery	Trying to be all things to all people. Falling back on familiar service-delivery approaches.
Staffing	Staff from other agencies bringing preconceptions.
Targeting	Trying to serve everyone.
Cost and budgeting	Depending too much on outside funding.
Evaluation	Measuring only inputs, not outputs.

As you design your collaboration, you will need to make important decisions in several areas: leadership and management (who's in charge), location of services (school-based or school-linked), delivery of services (which services, when, and where), staffing (new or reassigned), targeting (who are the clients), funding, and evaluation. In other words, you need to figure out what the collaboration will look like and how it will operate.

Who's in Charge?

Linking the services of several agencies with the school is a complex task. Just setting up services within a school is hard enough, but adding 5 to 10 other agencies with their own sets of rules, norms, and funding constraints can be daunting. One of the first things you'll need to do, therefore, is figure out how to manage the collaboration. It won't run itself; somebody will have to set goals, establish priorities, make decisions about which services to include, supervise and hire staff, and so on. The accounting firm Coopers & Lybrand found that of the time top management spends on developing partnerships and joint ventures, half is used to create them. One quarter is spent in planning and only 8 percent goes toward setting up the management system (Kanter 1992).

What kinds of committees or councils will you need and what will their functions be? Will you need to create new positions? Whatever approach you take, avoid the temptation to form more committees and subcommittees and have more meetings. The comedian Milton Berle is said to have observed that a committee is a group that takes minutes and loses hours. That doesn't mean that committees and meetings are a bad idea—you will need some structure—but bureaucracies tend to grow until they eventually collapse under their own weight. Some busy people will drop out if they don't see action. In one collaboration I worked with, an agency representative commented, "As far as I can see, all those people do is sit in meetings." He didn't stay involved much longer.

Policy Level

First, identify the primary governance and management functions that need to be carried out and who—or what group—can best carry them out. These will vary from one collaboration to another, but there are some basic functions you'll need to cover. Who, in each agency, has decision-making authority to enter into agreements, allocate funds, and hire staff? These top-level administrators—the buck-stoppers—will need to be involved. Call it the executive committee, governing board, or oversight committee; this group should set policy and decide on funding and governance questions. They not only need to have authority, they should also be in tune with the vision for the collaboration.

Walbridge Caring Communities in St. Louis, Missouri, set up a local advisory board made up of parents, school staff, community leaders, and agency representatives (Melaville and Blank 1993). In California's Healthy Start initiative, 80 percent of the collaborations set up an executive committee or council (Wagner, Shaver, Newman, Wechsler, Kelley, and Golan 1994).

Melaville and Blank (1993) warn that you shouldn't let one partner assume control of the group either by choice or default. Instead, strive for "shared leadership." If the school or district falls into this trap, for example, the other partners will come to think of the collaborative as the school's project and reduce their investment and commitment. Some collaborations have tried to rotate or share administrative positions. New Beginnings in San Diego, California, for example, splits the administrative positions between the Department of Social Services and the San Diego City Schools.

This high-level group of agency heads is important because they have decision-making power in their agencies. Without their buy-in, progress will be very slow—if there's any progress at all. They don't need to be involved in the day-to-day management of the collaboration. Events will creep along at a snail's pace if you wait for their input. The key to managing the executive committee is to use their time as efficiently as possible. Executives typically have busy calendars and if they don't believe the time they give to the collaboration is well-spent, they will back off.

"Meetings must be well organized and productive; tasks must be clearly articulated. Otherwise, members may stop coming, send subordinates, or drop out completely." (U.S. Department of Housing and Urban Development 1988, p. 6). Keep committee members informed of the initiative's progress through monthly status reports or memos from the collaboration director so they know the effect of their decisions.

Management Level

Someone also has to be responsible for the ongoing management of the collaboration and report to the policy-setting group. One option is to form a working group/action team of agency staff and mid-level administrators to meet weekly or biweekly to review progress and discuss problems.

Instead of forming a new committee for each issue, try to build on existing councils, networks, or other groups. This approach is recommended to new Healthy Start sites in California (California Department of Education 1994). If your combined budgets allow, you can hire a separate administrator to coordinate sites and agencies and report to the policy group. The collaboration director reports to the executive committee, monitors budgets, hires and supervises staff, lines up training programs, secures additional funding, represents the collaboration at meetings, links with the community, gets written commitments from other agencies, and works with the evaluator. You may still need someone else to manage the individual service site(s). Most have found that managing more than a few school-linked centers places unrealistic demands on a supervisor. One of the touchiest issues you'll deal with is that of on-site reporting relationships. Site directors will be set up for failure if they don't have some authority over staff.

Connecting with Others

Another important function is to keep all participating agencies up-to-date about what's going on in the collaboration and in the other agencies. Good communication will strengthen the collaboration and may lead to new connections and service-delivery options. You'll want to do what you can to ensure the involvement of all participating agencies and maximize each one's contribution. You will also probably want to craft interagency agreements that spell out the rights and obligations of each partner.

School-Based or School-Linked?

The first inclination of most collaborations is to put a family center for services at the school. There are several good arguments for doing that. Gangster Willie Sutton robbed banks because, "That's where the money is." Services should be at schools because that's where the kids are. Moreover, families are familiar with the site, teachers, and other staff. Just as important is that teachers, who are in daily contact with children, are in a position to know something of the problems their students may be encountering. The school also represents a central location and can often provide facilities for a family center, such as a classroom or portable building. Establishing a site here will make communication between collaboration staff and the school more convenient. Designating it a "collaboration" site gives the collaboration an identity. Finally, schools have a history of offering health and other noneducational services, and these can be extended or modified as agencies join each other to improve the service system (Levy and Shepardson 1992). Whether your collaborative operates at a single site or several, decisions about the location of services will be among the most important ones your group makes.

There are good arguments against school-based services, and these also must be considered. First, school enrollment boundaries frequently don't match those of the community or the other agencies involved. If a geographic definition is used to select eligible clients, then you'll need to decide if you're serving the children and parents from the school or those from the entire neighborhood. Low-income families tend to move often, frequently crossing school enrollment boundaries, and their children are transferred from school to school. Generally, though, they stay within the same community or neighborhood. For this reason, a community recreation center or other agency might be a more appropriate location for a family center than the school.

Second, placing services at the school doesn't ensure the participation of teachers and other staff. In fact, the close proximity can even breed suspicion as teachers wonder about what the social and health workers are doing and why they follow different work rules. Social workers' contracts may be structured so that they get "comp" time for work after regular hours, while whatever extra time teachers put in comes out of their own hide. Melding these two cultures can be a challenge, and the collaboration should be aware of the potential for discord.

Third, the parents you're most interested in involving may not have much affection for schools and what they represent. They're probably the same ones who are reluctant to come to parent-teacher conferences and never show up at open house. It's unlikely they're nostalgic for their high school "happy days." If this is the case for a large number of parents, then some other location in the community might be more appropriate. In Reno, Nevada, for example, the Children's Cabinet has its own building where counseling and other services are offered. It also has satellite centers near key schools.

A fourth possible drawback of school-based services is the potential for conflict over authority at the school site. In other words, "Who's in charge?" School-site administrators are used to being the sole authority at their site. What happens when they have to share it? Or when there are staff on-site (e.g., from other agencies) not under their supervision? Work out issues of management in advance or at least have them in mind when the collaboration starts up. Relationships are key.

In choosing a site for collaborative services, try to find one that is easy to reach and where families and children feel comfortable. You want to give families better access to services, so ask them where they would like to receive them. Don't just rely on what you and your partners think. For example, if space is readily available at a recreation center, investigate whether it's really the best place to house a family center. Maybe the space is available because it's inconvenient for families to get there.

In designing the services you offer, you'll need to decide on the types of services at your center and who will offer them. In other words, you'll need to define your product. Collaborations typically offer a range of prevention, support, and crisis intervention services organized by level of intensity, from short, information-and-referral assistance to long-term case management. What your collaboration offers will of course depend on the needs of the children and their families as well as the resources of you and your partners. As you plan, keep in mind that you don't need to offer everything and not everything has to be concentrated at one site.

Levels of Service

Much of the literature on integrated services describes three levels of service: information and referral, on-site prevention and support, and case management (e.g., Melaville and Blank 1993). It will be useful to consider these levels as you flesh out the design of your collaboration.

Information and referral can help students or other family members find their way to services not provided at the family center. Many families could better navigate the existing system if they simply knew more about what help was available and where to get it. The service center can be a repository of such information.

On-site prevention and support services might include child care, counseling, literacy assistance, youth development, and mentoring. Education and training for students, adults, or outstationed staff from other agencies might also be offered. Other services could be case review panels, case conferences, or student review teams that bring together teachers, counselors, nurses, and other school and agency staff to review cases of troubled children.

Case management connects families with a tailored set of prevention, support, and crisis-intervention and treatment services. Multiple providers establish agreements to accept referrals and provide priority services to families who need assistance beyond what is directly offered at the center. On-site staff will typically assess family strengths and needs and then work with the family to develop a family service plan, which may include any number of services and connections to services. The case manager will then be responsible for monitoring the family's progress over time and checking in periodically with the child or key family member. For the neediest families, this might mean very close contact and support for the first few weeks or months, including periodic home visits. When the family members become comfortable with the services and agencies involved—if they do—the intensity of support from the case manager is reduced. This outline of case management assumes a focus on the family or child as a treatment or service unit. In that way, the services are family-focused and more integrated.

A Services Road Map

Think about how you'd like services in the community to look from the perspective of the family or child. As they encounter your services, is it clear to them what to do next and where to go? If you don't know, they certainly won't. Develop a flow chart that clearly identifies the route clients take from the first encounter to the day their case is closed. You will need to specify the source of referrals, intake and assessment procedures, service plan development, service assignment, and staff responsibility.

The source of referrals might be a teacher, the child or family member, school staff, or staff from other agencies. Teachers need to be trained in what to refer for and trained in how to make referrals. If they don't fully understand the purpose of the collaborative, then students might be sent to the family center for the wrong reasons. A teacher might assume, for example, that the collaboration is for disciplining students who act out in class, even though this responsibly still lies with the school administration.

Strive to develop a single point of intake and assessment. This will simplify matters not only for your customers, but for you as well. It will keep them from running all over town trying to find the help they need, and it will allow you to efficiently and uniformly assess and assist families in need. Work with other agencies to see if you can develop common application procedures.

Staffing

Who will staff the center? Will you hire new staff or use reassigned workers from other agencies? Will they be existing employees with redefined roles? The collaboration will need to be clear about reporting relationships and responsibilities. What are the reporting relationships? If the site director is manager, does he or she manage the staff from another agency, or do staff answer to their supervisor at the home agency?

Consider New Beginnings in San Diego. At an elementary school site, staff from partner agencies were reassigned to act as case managers called family service advocates (FSAs). They left behind their agency roles and took on any number of tasks to meet the needs of participating families, from counseling to brokering assistance from their parent agencies or others. They were no longer Child Protective Services (CPS) caseworkers, school counselors, or JOBS workers. Instead, each assumed the more varied (and less-structured) job of family service advocate. Supplementing the FSAs were a nurse practitioner and other staff (Melaville and Blank 1993, New Beginnings Team 1990).

Other collaborations have chosen to relocate staff but maintain their basic job functions. Staff from CPS continue to handle the CPS issues and the AFDC person sticks with income maintenance. In Phoenix, Arizona, for instance, the Department of Economic Security relocated a "unit" of more than 20 workers to a site on school district grounds; job descriptions remained the same. Others have relied on volunteers. This approach is sometimes called colocation, and can involve individual staff as well as entire units.

A third option is to hire new staff. This is seldom possible without outside funding, such as a state grant. New Jersey's School-Based Youth Services Program and the Family Resource Centers in Kentucky are based on state grant systems that allow each local collaborative to recruit staff. In practice, you may hire the same staff anyway, but the procedures they follow will probably be different.

You will face at least two major challenges in regard to staffing. First will be the task of getting staff to assume new, more flexible roles. Whether they're former income-maintenance workers or school counselors, taking on the new assignment in a collaboration will involve a change in professional norms and culture. Instead of following the prescribed rules they are accustomed to, staff will need to see how they can work with families, not just individuals. It may be difficult not to divide clients by problem, and to address families as a whole. Home visits may not be part of the professional experience of staff, and some may be uncomfortable entering the homes of clients. Mitchell and Scott (1994) suggest that staff from case-oriented agencies, such as social services, are accustomed to defining their job status by the number of cases. When the number of cases is reduced, they may feel their status has been diminished.

Give your staff adequate support and the training they need. As Gardner observes, "A social services worker relocated to a school is often coming to a less safe environment, doing an unfamiliar job, with fewer rules and routines, and on an unfamiliar team. This is a worker who needs more than the usual level of support and rewards" (1994, pp.192-193). I'll say more about professional development later.

A second big challenge will be to build relationships between your staff and the school. Because classroom teachers are in frequent contact with students—your primary clients—they need to be familiar with the purpose and design of the collaboration. They will also be an important source of referrals and might also be a tremendous help for those students in their classes. Be aware that the teachers and the collaboration staff are going to see each other differently because they come from different professional cultures. You might encounter professional resentment from teachers about the flexibility allowed case managers and their freedom to come and go. They will also learn of contract differences that allow social services workers "comp" time for extra hours worked, while they receive none. On the other side, collaboration staff may feel left out of the school culture and activities. Involve teachers in meetings or other activities so they can come to understand the purpose of the collaboration. Social service and health staff can learn more about the school by participating in "child study teams" or other school committees. In some schools, the collaboration staff regularly attend teachers' meetings, sometimes giving a brief report on their own activities and progress.

Before you select staff, explore with the team how staff might be acquired in ways most compatible with your vision. Costs and other practical factors, such as availability of qualified workers, may eventually determine what you end up with, but try for your most ambitious design anyway. Brainstorm with the frontline staff to see what you can come up with. Then, try to get the right to choose which staff will be reassigned from partner agencies. If that's not possible, at least try to have a voice in who will be working in the collaboration, especially if you're operating a pilot. The pilot activity will be under the scrutiny of the top managers and funders, and you want to ensure you have the best staffing possible, not just the most eager or flexible.

Finally, avoid getting all the staff from the same agency, such as CPS or even social services. It's better to have a mix; otherwise the temptation to revert to old ways will be very strong. It won't be easy. You will not only have to deal with greater differences in work habits and culture, but also with the fact that success will be jointly measured across agencies (Gardner 1994).

Staff Development

The systems you're trying to link up—school, social service, and health—have their own unique sets of operating procedures, rules and regulations, language, and professional norms. They aren't used to working with each other in ways that involve sharing responsibility or clients. Your staff will need to learn about each other's agencies and how the staffs can work together. They need to know about the partner agencies policies and practices. They'll also need to learn about community resources, clinical and service delivery, case documentation and record keeping, and the concepts of positive youth development and family support (Center for the Future of Children 1992, Melaville and Blank 1991). An investment in effective training early in the collaboration's history will pay off in the long run.

Of course, the kind of staff development you provide will depend on how your collaboration is organized and on the staff you're using. Most will have come from agencies that promote competition among staff rather than cooperation and consensus building (Melaville and Blank

1991). If you have reassigned staff from partner agencies, it's essential that they learn about the new ways of working. How much their job description changes will affect the training. If you've organized your initiative around "family advocates" or "case mangers" then their responsibilities may be very different from what they were in their parent institution. In some collaborations, the primary functions of workers remain fairly consistent with their earlier job (e.g., an income maintenance worker from social services is assigned to the family center to improve access to families). For those workers, the amount of cross-training may be less than when the worker has an entirely new job description, such as a family advocate. There, the increased autonomy and discretion in how to work with families may be demanding for staff.

In many ways, good collaboration comes down to developing relationships—with families, with other staff, and across agencies. Effective staff support will foster ways for case mangers or other staff to learn better how to work together and how to connect with counterparts in referral agencies. As Bruner (1991) points out, formal agreements ultimately are played out as staff talking to staff and working out ways to help a family in need.

A final point about staff development concerns record keeping and documentation. There's a lot of pressure on collaborations to demonstrate their value, from communities, funders, and sponsoring agencies. Documentation and evaluation have to rely on the frontline worker to capture a lot of the information on families. Don't be surprised if your staff are not used to keeping accurate and complete records. Some, such as social workers, will be accustomed to keeping case notes, but in a fairly unstructured way. Social services eligibility workers will be more comfortable with numerical, check-off data. Still others won't have kept any records in their previous jobs.

Be careful that your data-collection system doesn't become so elaborate that the site staff spend more time keeping up with paperwork than working with families. We are all eager to know everything that's happening with collaborations, but, as is pointed out in the section on evaluation below, you can only deal with a certain amount of information at a time. You'll need to work out a system that allows you and the evaluator to get needed information, but not at the expense of the case managers' mental health. Too much paperwork drives them crazy. Assess their experience with paperwork and try to reach a balance between valuable documentation and time with families.

Targeting

Who are the customers? As services are made available, the collaboration will need to decide who to include as clients. To some, the answer to this question might seem obvious—serving the kids enrolled in our school and their families. Some collaborations, like Project Pride in West Joliet, Illinois, concentrate on special populations, such as high school girls whose families receive Aid to Families with Dependent Children (AFDC) (Levy and Shepardson, 1992). In collaborations that colocate programs, who the clients are may be partly determined by the eligibility rules of participating agencies. These could include residence requirements. Thus, in this case, anyone in a particular area who qualifies for any of the agencies' services can be served by the collaboration.

Targeting can be made along a variety of dimensions: geography, age, school or other program enrollment, or intensity of need. The Murphy Family Center in Phoenix, Arizona, for example, used area of residence as a targeting criterion. A unit of the Department of Economic Security (DES) was relocated to the school district and made services available to anyone living in the zip-code area which almost matches the school district's enrollment area. Mitchell and Scott (1994) believe that because recent initiatives have redefined eligible clients in terms of geographic area rather than unique client problems, they have reduced the fragmentation common in the system.

Once you begin to offer more intensive interventions like case management, the demand on staff will become a consideration. Even scheduling case reviews can multiply the time commitments of your staff and those of the school. At some point, you may have to admit you can't serve everyone. On one hand, having a surplus of customers will validate the collaboration and demonstrate its need to agency heads and other potential skeptics. On the other, it's hard to make choices about whom to serve. In taking a preventive approach, you might first decide to focus on students in kindergarten through grade 2. Once your family center is in operation, however, the collaboration might find it difficult to deny services to older students and their families.

Workers will need to balance their case loads with the demand for services. If counselors and other staff are spread too thin, the quality of services will suffer. An appropriate case load will depend on the services provided. Income maintenance workers may be accustomed to having hundreds of clients for what they call case management. More intensive work may mean a maximum case load of 20. Ultimately, the standard for a realistic case load will depend on the design of the services and the culture of the organizations involved.

If you don't define who the clients are, then, in a very real sense, the demand for services will eventually resolve the targeting issue for you. Those at the head of the waiting list will get served and those at the end will not, even though they might need services more (Gardner 1992). It's up to you to determine whether you want to make a deliberate choice about who's eligible—or let the numbers decide.

Dialing for Dollars

Funding is one of the hardest things for new (and even established) collaboratives to deal with. In smaller, less ambitious initiatives, costs may not be a worry, but once you start to redesign services, move staff around, or occupy separate space, you'll need to think about how you're going to pay for things. The fact that state and federal funding sources are in a state of flux (e.g., welfare reform) doesn't make things easier. But at least some seem to be going in a direction favorable to comprehensive and integrated services. Regulations are presumably being reduced and streamlined to make it easier for schools and other agencies to receive support for collaborative work. Funding is also the single issue most likely to divide collaboration members. As Farrow and Joe (1992) point out, everyone is in favor of integrating their services and working together until you start asking how to pay for it. This "puts their commitment to the test" (Farrow and Joe 1992, p. 57).

In the present fiscal climate, it's a good idea to count on little or no extra funding. If you are lucky enough to get some start-up grant money, then so much the better. That can help you get off on the right foot and allow you to try out some things at the beginning. Your long-term focus, however, should be on more stable sources.

Tapping federal and state program dollars is an increasingly popular strategy for financing school-linked services. In the education, social services, and health sectors, money is available. Within education, funding possibilities range from your own state and local general-education fund to categorical money through Title 1 (Chapter 1), special education, and others. Title 1 legislation has recently made it clear that you can pay for connecting services with the school, even if the school is not operating a schoolwide program. Social services options include Title IV-B of the Social Security Act and the Family Support Act (JOBS) program. Health support is primarily through Medicaid, which includes the Early and Periodic Screening, Diagnosis, and Treatment (EPSDT) program. Medicaid also provides a wide range of services and programs designed to assist pregnant women and young children. States have the freedom to specify eligibility and coverage (Kirst 1993), and several are looking at ways that collaborations can qualify for some of these resources. Another option is to link up with a qualified Medicaid provider, such as a hospital, that can offer reimbursable services as part of the collaboration. Alternatively, EPSDT can be used to pay for some special-education services, case management, outreach, screening, and health prevention (Kirst 1993).

Even with the impending overhauls at the federal level, these sources will still be around, but they probably won't get much simpler. Compared to social services and health, educational funding streams are a piece of cake. As Farrow and Joe warn, "The degree of reporting, documentation, and eligibility scrutiny differs widely from source to source. By the time the funding stream reaches a community, the stream consists of a confusing and inaccessible array of funding 'opportunities' that very few people understand" (Farrow and Joe 1992, p. 60). You're going to need your partners' help on this one. Together, you will have to track new legislation and figure out the eligibility and record-keeping requirements of these programs. These requirements may in turn have implications for how your school-linked services are designed—if you don't meet the requirements, you won't get the funding (Kirst 1993).

The Weaning Process

Several options are available for start-up money; in fact, many collaborations have begun simply because They're following the money. Schools and other agencies hear about a grant program and get together to prepare their response to the request for proposals. This has been the case in California, Kentucky, New Jersey, and other states. If your state or local government dangles a grant in front of you, go for it. Remember, though, that you can't rely on special funding indefinitely. Unless you find a way to make your collaboration self-supporting, much of your hard work will be lost. A key argument for integrating services, after all, is to provide a more efficient and cost-effective way of delivering services. While start-up funds are important, maybe even essential, you need to shoot for eventual self-sufficiency. Otherwise, when the grant runs out, many of your partners will scurry back to their home agencies.

Evaluation: Achieving Accountability

A complex interagency collaboration, with many different services and a varied group of clients, presents a formidable challenge for an evaluator. In fact, the field of evaluating interagency collaborations is still developing and there are few models to draw upon. Nevertheless, an emerging collaboration is making a mistake if it doesn't put some time into planning and paying for an evaluation that will tell the members how they are doing and what effect they are having on children and their families.

There are several practical reasons to invest in an evaluation. First, what happens to clients both during and following service is information programs should use to improve the services they provide. This information is not simply something to provide to administrators or funders.

Without this knowledge, programs operate more on faith and assumptions than on facts. Better data can mean better services. Information on referral completion (did the client make and keep an appointment at the referred agency?), can tell staff whether they need to follow up more directly on referrals—or even accompany clients as part of the process. Information on students' school enrollment status and attendance can help a case manager identify who needs more attention. A mark of a good evaluation is the extent to which it can be used by the program being evaluated.

Second, funding for a collaboration will be based more and more on the documentation of client outcomes—not just on services performed. Far too many evaluations are still focused on inputs instead of outcomes, on the number of "service units" rather than on what happens to participants. Both government and foundation funding now tend to support efforts that demonstrate not only the number of services delivered, but also proof that they are producing a positive effect for clients. Without data on outcomes, the funders are unable to tell whether the collaboration or its component programs are meeting their specified goals: they know only that they are fulfilling their contractual obligations and providing services to the targeted populations.

For example, as part of a collaboration, a local community provides gang prevention counseling to 50 teenagers on a six-month cycle. The stated goals of this activity are that youth will stay out of the juvenile justice system, stay in school, improve (school) attendance, or reenter school. Simply reporting the number of students receiving counseling tells us nothing about whether the behavior of any of the clients changed during or after the community center's intervention. Do they join gangs? Stay in school? Have they been arrested? What is their attendance record? Without outcome reporting, it is difficult to tell if the program is working well.

Clarify Your Purposes

In order to be clear about an evaluation, the collaboration leaders first need to clarify their own purposes. What do you want the evaluation to tell you? Is the primary purpose to measure the outcomes of the program for administrators, the policy board, and funders? Is it to identify problems and test out alternatives for staff? Suggest improvements in program design and operation? Determine if the initiative is working as planned?

Within the goals of the collaboration any number of objectives might be identified. These could range from educational achievement for children to community safety. A successful evaluation does not depend on the number of objectives included, but on the selection of objectives that might reasonably be achieved and that can be measured. Revisit the goals and objectives in your vision statement once more to ensure that they meet these criteria.

Define achievable goals and objectives

The collaboration should be able to make a logical argument for why and how the program can realistically bring about each outcome. For example, your first goal might be to improve the educational success of children and youth. Is it reasonable to expect that the services you offer (tutoring, counseling) will have a significant effect on student achievement? Be realistic. If the goals and objectives are too ambitious or only indirectly related to the collaboration's efforts, you will almost certainly fail to meet them. You may have some broader goals, such as improving school climate or the community environment. For goals like these, it is critical that you come up with clear definitions of "school climate" and "community environment" and how they might be affected by the services you provide. Be careful to assess how what you are doing affects indicators such as the juvenile crime rate in the school, catchment area, or housing.

Consider, for example, the gang prevention counseling and case management program mentioned earlier. It is unlikely the counseling and advocacy the community center provides will have a significant effect on student achievement. A more realistic expectation is that the gang prevention will help youth stay out of the juvenile justice system, enroll in school, and show improved school attendance. That's where you should look for outcomes.

Improved data gathering, reporting, and analysis will require an investment of time and energy at both the program and collaboration level. To some program staff,

45

that means taking away from the services they provide. As one agency's executive director once pleaded with me, "Don't make the data collection too intrusive." These are valid concerns, and you should explore ways to collect the needed information without taking too much staff time. For instance, the collaboration should make sure that only essential data are being gathered; if data will not be used, why collect them?

Another important consideration in selecting objectives is the time in which change might be expected. It might be impossible to meet long-term goals during the time of the evaluation, but certain interim indicators should be identified. How do you show "improved health," for example? An increase in the number of dental examinations doesn't exactly demonstrate improved health, but it points in that direction.

A final point about goals and objectives is that the evaluation should be flexible enough to identify and measure the effects of short-term, targeted services offered in specialized programs. If the program at one school implements an in-school suspension program, for example, then data on attendance, tardy arrival, or homework completion for those students might be calculated separately to determine the effect of the special program. If successful, the program can be extended to other sites.

Select measurable indicators

Second, be sure that the objectives are measurable and data for measuring them can be obtained. As part of this process, the evaluator should be able to specify *for each indicator*:

- The clients for whom outcomes are expected (all eligible clients? families? high school students?).
- The source of data (intake forms, school information, surveys, interviews).
- How and when the data are gathered.

Specify Clients for Whom Outcomes Are Expected

Make sure you know for whom outcomes are expected. If one goal is educational success, for example, the evaluation must be careful to match academic achievement data to program participants who received academic assistance. While an argument can be made that improved health and self-esteem will be reflected in academic achievement, the connection is indirect and most likely long-term. For secondary school students, GPA or enrollment in college preparation classes might be better indicators than standardized test scores. It wouldn't be feasible to administer a standardized test and, given the current status of state assessments, schools may not have any such data. At the elementary level, assignment to Chapter 1 or special education classes might be better measures to consider. Whatever indicator is selected, it is important to work with the schools to determine what is appropriate and available.

One useful alternative is to collect information on a small sample of clients that shows their experiences in the program and the effects of these experiences on them. Case studies of individual clients can in some ways be more powerful than statistical descriptions of program effects. Interviews with 10 to 12 clients from one of the programs about the intervention they received, their impressions of the services, and changes they might have made in their attitudes or behavior can be an effective way of explaining and demonstrating possible program effects. While clients might not be able to articulate specific changes in behavior, the interviewer can elicit useful information through direct questions, (e.g., "How many times have you been absent from school this week?"). If clients are followed over the course of the intervention and in follow-up interviews a few months later, changes in their behavior can be adequately captured.

Remember the Evaluator's Question and How to Answer It

The critical question in an evaluation of a social program is whether the program effects are different from what would have occurred without the intervention or with an alternative intervention. The challenge for the evaluator is to find a way to answer that question so that the findings are plausible. Because program evaluations take place in the real world and not in a laboratory, designing an evaluation becomes a process of making adjustments to reality. Random assignment of subjects to experimental and control groups is rarely possible in real-world evaluations. Nevertheless, meaningful and useful results can still be obtained.

There are several key elements of the evaluation that you need to consider, in addition to those having to do with goals and objectives. These include:

- comparison groups
- data sources and collection procedures
- data analysis and reporting

Comparison groups. Comparisons are essential to an evaluation of program impact, and the plausibility of evaluation results depends largely on the way those comparisons are made. In evaluating social programs, randomly assigning subjects into experimental and control groups is seldom feasible. This does not mean that we can't make meaningful comparisons. Instead, try to think of other possibilities, such as these:

- Within-school comparisons (unserved but eligible students matched on critical variables).
- Comparisons with the total school population (e.g., high school attendance rate).
- Comparisons with Human Services data if appropriate matches are technically possible.
- Samples of students drawn from other schools with similar student populations.
- Retrospective or "lagged" comparisons (cohorts from prior years).

Data sources and collection procedures. Several sources of data are possible: data already collected by the schools or other agencies, data collected from intake and other collaboration forms, and surveys and interviews created by the evaluator. For goals that concern health or family functioning, the evaluation should also consider the kinds of records that might be available at county or state social services agencies. If program clients could be matched with the county data, then several realistic indicators might be available. Another key source is the data routinely kept by the collaboration programs or the school, for example, visits to a doctor, visits to the family center for health reasons, a regular source of medical care, or absences for health reasons. Decreases in these would indicate progress in improving children's health.

The kinds of data and specific procedures for gathering them need to be negotiated with those responsible for potential data sources, such as the family advocates, schools, or social services. Dates for data collection (once per semester, annually, each grading period) and the agency responsible (evaluator, school, family advocates) must also be established. Unless a clear agreement is reached about who is gathering and reporting each type of data and at what time, data collection will not be successful. The evaluator should create a table that specifies the following:

- indicators
- subjects (clients)
- comparisons
- data sources/measurement tools
- collection responsibility
- frequency of data collection

Data analysis and reporting. Data analysis strategies are an essential part of the evaluation plan and should be specified as much as possible in advance. Analyses will be both qualitative and quantitative. For the qualitative analysis (e.g., of case studies), decide which data sources are going to be used and what procedures will be for data reduction, summary, comparison, and interpretation. While the particular patterns, themes, or categories that might emerge from the data cannot be known in advance, the data to be examined and the analysis procedures can be decided.

Quantitative analyses can be largely descriptive. In other words, they will rely on frequencies and percentages, rather than on statistical tests of significance. Determine which variables will be analyzed and the relationships among them that will be explored. Analyses should be designed so they show relationships among different groups and disaggregate data by important independent variables (program enrollment, demographics). Achievement of objectives such as school attendance, for example, should be reported by grade, ethnicity, and services received for both collaboration students and comparison groups.

Another purpose of the analyses is to assess program improvement. It might be useful to know, for example, how many of the clients referred for jobs also received gang prevention counseling. A key issue for collaboration should be the integration of services across agencies and programs, and data analysis should be designed to capture examples of clients who are served by multiple programs.

4
Staying Alive and Going to Scale

LET'S ASSUME YOU'VE STARTED A COLLABORATION, SUCH AS A FAMILY center at a school, and are serving children and families from the neighborhood. As you look toward the future, one of three things can happen. First, you can maintain your collaborative's current scope, continuing to solidify and strengthen your services and connections. Or you might begin to build on your success, expanding to other sites and into the larger community. In the jargon of reformers, you could "go to scale." A final possibility is that your initiative is discontinued for lack of funding, support, or interest. In this final chapter, let's look at how you can ensure the first, work toward the second, and avoid the third—all at the same time.

Staying Alive

If you want your collaboration to last, it's a good idea to start with a pilot that focuses on one neighborhood and the agencies that work there (Guthrie and Guthrie 1991, Melaville and Blank 1993). This prototype will help those involved to know the families in the area, their needs, and the barriers they face in getting access to services. Partner agencies will also get to know each other and work out kinks in policies and agreements, even though the resource commitment from each may be relatively small. Finally, you can learn from the experience of trying out your vision of collaboration in a real-life setting. This is what you need when and if you're ready to expand to other sites and communities (Melaville and Blank 1993).

To get things going on a small scale, you don't need the complete involvement of everyone or each agency. As Fullan suggests in relation to school reform, you do need a core group of people who can initiate the effort, begin to show success, and build momentum (1992). He says to start small, think big, and "maintain a bias for action"—learn by doing (1992, p. 91). If a key partner, such as the health department, appears lukewarm on the idea of collaboration, don't insist they be involved at first. If you do, you might open yourself up to potential sabotage—collaboration can be very threatening. Initiate what you and your active, committed partners can, and continue to coax the more reluctant ones. Even if the skeptics drop out, keep them informed about positive developments with mailings, newsletters, and such. Chances are that as you begin to demonstrate the advantages of working together, they'll come around.

School-linked services advocates tend to press practitioners toward expansion, advising them to go to scale as soon as possible (Melaville and Blank 1993). Some gurus, no doubt, are driven by their enthusiasm for reform and consider anything less than a total transformation of the system as tantamount to failure. Moreover, a natural tendency among "change masters"—like you—is to try to keep one eye on the pilot project and the other on a larger dissemination effort. That's not only physically hard to do, programmatically it is also difficult. Another problem is the tendency of top- and mid-level managers to get "over-committee'd." As each new site forms its oversight committee or governing board, there are only so many "governors" or "overseers" to go around in the county or jurisdiction. When engaged in something as complex as school-linked services, you should resist the temptation to expand until you are ready. Make sure you can demonstrate success before starting to expand, and don't take away valuable resources to add other sites.

You will inevitably be drawn into the larger system, anyway, so don't force it. In the meantime, concentrate on providing the best services for children and families. Refine the service delivery design you've set up, solidify relationships with partner agencies and the community, and document the successes you've had (evaluate). Support those who directly work with children and families. Provide them the time, freedom, and training they need to flourish. It's in the day-to-day interactions and delivery of services to children and families that your initiative will rise or fall.

At some point, however, you'll start looking beyond the narrow confines of your collaborative. You will come into contact with other schools or communities interested in experimenting with integrating services. Some will contact you, and you may have more requests for visits or consultation than you can handle. New Beginnings, for instance, had to restrict the days visitors could tour its facility. In addition, as the program matures, a ripple effect will inevitably lead you to barriers associated with state, local, and federal regulations and policies. Your search for opportunities for continued funding will also take you in the direction of the larger system.

Going to Scale

Even a collaboration that involves a single school, or only part of a community, ultimately depends upon the larger system for survival. Eventually, it may be difficult to sustain it as an add-on program or pilot. Suppose, for example, you have reassigned staff from one or more agencies to work in a family center. This may work well in the short run, but gradually you'll be drawn into a larger context. You then may come to see your own fledgling initiative as "tinkering around the edges" and begin to consider expanding to other sites.

So what's involved in going to scale? Unfortunately, that's something we don't have much experience with. As Melaville and Blank (1993) admit, "As yet, no jurisdictions have gone to scale or developed an explicit strategy for achieving that end" (p. 78). Bob Slavin makes a similar point in relation to spreading educational innovations when he says the research "is so much a documentation of failure that it's hard to know what to make of it" (Olson 1994, p. 43). Policymakers are hungry for information on successful models and how to go to scale (McCart 1993). Expansion is not a matter of replication, cookie-cutter style, but developing the context for change. Moreover, there's strong evidence to suggest that real change isn't linear. One idea of systemic reform, for example, suggests that national educational success will occur if states align their curriculum, professional development, assessments, and resources with the high standards for student learning captured in the national and state goals (Olson 1994). Others say this reasoning is flawed. To paraphrase George Bernard Shaw, you can't change society by "brute sanity" (Fullan 1992).

Bear in mind that going to scale will not be easy and will take time and money. It's impossible to estimate how much it might cost. Specific, single-focus innovations take at least a couple of years to get up and running. More complex, institutional change may require 5-10 years (Fullan 1992). Be prepared for the long haul.

Talk of scaling up has spread in the past couple of years. As for "how to," we're only a little further along than we were in the '80s. Still, the experiences of education reformers and school-linked services efforts help point us in directions that make sense. Initiating school-linked services is harder than educational reforms because you're dealing with multiple agencies and a larger number of bureaucracies and egos. Nevertheless, there are some principles you can follow that should lead toward a successful spread of interagency collaboration. What seems to make a difference in getting people and institutions to change is for them to organize their efforts around a few "powerful themes" (Fullan, 1992). I see successful expansion coming with two complementary approaches: (1) a focus on capacity-building, and (2) support of professional development.

Focus on Capacity-Building

To spread from a single, interagency collaboration site, you will need to build the capacity in other communities to support the development of change. The cookie-cutter replication approach to scaling up is now largely discredited. In education, we used to think that you could buy a program off the shelf and stick it in any classroom; now we know better. Unless the classroom is ready—and that means teacher, principal, and larger context—there's little chance the innovation will take hold. Most reformers now realize that change occurs on a case-by-case basis and depends on local interest, commitment, and capacities. As Fullan (1992) says:

> Assume that changing the culture of institutions is the real agenda, not implementing particular innovations. Put another way, when implementing particular innovations, we should always pay attention to whether the institution is developing or not (p. 107).

Capacity-building means creating a vision, developing local leadership, and fostering buy-in. Just as in your own collaboration, the first step is to create a vision. In new settings, the challenge is to help people come up with their own vision of where they can go—their collaboration and how to get there. Concentrate on features of your collaboration or other prominent ones, emphasizing a few key principles and strategies. Continuously compare them to the local situation, checking the fit and exploring how things might be done to bring about the ends they seek.

New sites will also need local leadership if they're to succeed. That means using staff in lead agencies who have the interest, credibility, and time to bring off an interagency effort. Bruner (1991) suggests that you furnish new sites with "resource change agents" who can help develop local leadership and build local strengths. You or your own staff might play this role on a limited basis. Research shows that change agents can be effective in stimulating and supporting local initiatives as part of a process of "mutual adaptation" (McLaughlin 1990). The important thing is how they interact with the local context, including the front-line deliverers of service.

Finally, you can build capacity through commitment and buy-ins from key constituents—schools, service agencies, and the community. Commitment has to start at the top, as well as through the kind of networking and sharing discussed below.

A common concern among the initiators of reform is how to maintain the integrity of what they have done and at the same time acknowledge that there will be some variation from place to place in the way a collaboration is administered and supported. You'll have to try not to be too concerned about "model drift"—where local adaptations don't appear to be truly collaborative in approach or designed to provide integrated services. Individual implementers will have to work out their own way of doing things. They need pressure to change, but ultimately have to decide for themselves. Plus, as Schorr points out, "community-proof" or "people-proof" programs in the field of human services are no more likely to emerge than "teacher-proof" curriculums. New sites must be allowed "to make it their own" (Schorr 1988, p. 276).

Professional Development

Everyone likes to talk nowadays about the uselessness of the one-shot workshop—even though I'd bet that it's still the most popular form of professional development in schools. People seem much less clear about what to replace it with. My vote goes for strategies that bring professionals together for sharing and networking. Some recent studies suggest that teachers and other school staff learn new practices most effectively when they have on-going access to colleagues to share and discuss experiences and ideas. Everything we know about institutional change suggests it's people-to-people connections that will make change happen, much more than what we tell them or give them to read. If, in your efforts to build the skills of administrators and staff in other sites, you only did one thing, it should be to foster the development of peer networks that provide more continuous opportunities for the exchange of ideas and experiences. Maybe you can build on existing networks created for a different or similar purpose, such as school improvement or restructuring networks and associations.

More formal training can come along with the establishment of networks, as occasional outside experts or consultants are brought to interact with network members. If, for example, the group decides that additional, in-depth information and training on case management is needed, then they can arrange for that to occur.

Demonstration sites can be an effective part of this approach. Your site, or other collaboratives, can host occasional visits from network members that allow those just starting out to see how a collaboration works in practice. It also gives those on-site a chance to get feedback from interested outsiders. Nothing can bring a group further in its development than to actually see the program in operation.

Networking and mutual site visits are also a way to engage those most critical to the success of the project. These include workers in day-to-day contact with children and their families—teachers, social workers, nurses, counselors, and others. They seldom are able to attend training sessions or conferences because of their on-site duties. Instead, administrators are the ones who benefit from more formal learning opportunities. Change strategies that rely on the connections between front-line staff may be more effective in the long run than the top-down approach specified by administrators and policymakers (McLaughlin 1990).

Conclusion

Some final suggestions for staying alive and going to scale: First, get smart about funding and legislation. The late '90s will be a time of dramatic change in social policy in this country, from welfare reform to the reinvention of government (Gore 1993, Osborne and Gaebler 1993). Find a way to monitor legislation and formulate responses to shifts in policy.

Second, get good at proposal writing. While the self-sufficient collaboration is a goal, additional support that grants can provide for staff development and expansion shouldn't be ignored or underestimated.

Finally, get accustomed to reporting your successes, especially ones that show cost-effectiveness. Don't expect to have reliable cost-effectiveness data, because you won't. Instead, uncover and report those stories where you've seen savings. As Schorr (1988) points out, measuring the savings from prevention is difficult, since, by definition, we expect the outcome of prevention to be nothing. On the other hand, some cost savings can be documented and reported, particularly around specific incidents. Take care to record and report these. Even the Perry Preschool data (Berrueta-Clement, Schweinhart, Barnett, Epstein, and Weikart 1984) can carry some weight, but more recent and locally significant information would be better.

In a discussion of school restructuring, Elmore (1990) suggests that the most likely scenario for educational reform for the '90s will be an "adaptive realignment" in which restructuring becomes part of larger change initiatives. He sees little likelihood for a wholesale transformation of the entire system based on the ideas of school restructuring. It is unrealistic, he says, because the social and political factors are too powerful. Trying to transform the way educational, social services, and health agencies serve children and families would seem to be an even more unrealistic undertaking. Elmore's notion of adaptive realignment can be applied to interagency collaboration as well.

In an adaptive realignment scenario, interagency collaboration comes to be recognized as at least a partial solution to larger societal problems, such as welfare, poverty, and crime. Without such social and political pressure, we're not likely to see a dramatic shift toward school-linked services. The sclerotic bureaucracies that house the services we're trying to link are expert at resisting change. The question, then, will be to see how well school-linked services advocates can attach this approach to the problems most prominent for society. Unless the community at large, and the agencies that serve it, see an advantage for adopting a school-linked services approach, then they won't do it. Key constituencies have to foresee tangible payoffs for themselves. Only when integrating services is recognized as a way to improve the responsiveness, efficiency, and cost of children's and family services will there be a real chance for large-scale implementation.

References

Berrueta-Clement, J.F., L.J. Schweinhart, W.S. Barnett, A.E. Epstein, and D. P. Weikart. (1984). *Changed Lives: The Effects of the Perry Preschool Programs on Youths through Age 19.* Ypsilanti, Mich.: High/Scope Press.

Bruner, C. (1991). *Thinking Collaboratively: Ten Questions and Answers to Help Policy Makers Improve Children's Services.* Education and Human Services Consortium. Washington, D.C.

Bruner, D., K. Bell, C. Brindis, H. Chang, and W. Scarbrough. (1993). *Charting a Course: Assessing a Community's Strengths and Needs.* Falls Church, Va.: National Center for Service Integration.

California Department of Education. (1994). *Request for Applications: Senate Bill 620 (Chapter 759, Statutes of 1991) The Healthy Start Support Services for Children Act.* Sacramento, Calif.: Author

Center for the Future of Children. (1992). "Analysis." *The Future of Children* 2, 2: 6-18.

Committee for Economic Development. (1985). *Investing in Our Children.* New York: Committee for Economic Development.

Deal, T.E., and A. A. Kennedy. (1982). *Corporate Cultures: The Rites and Rituals of Corporate Life.* Reading, Mass.: Addison-Wesley.

Elmore, D. (1990). "Conclusion." In *Restructuring Schools: The Next Generation of Educational Reform*, edited by D. Elmore. San Francisco: Jossey-Bass.

Farrow, F., and T. Joe. (1992). "Financing School-linked, Integrated Services." *The Future of Children* 2, 2: 56-67.

Fullan, M. G. (1992). *The New Meaning of Educational Change.* New York: Teachers College Press.

Gardner, S. (1992). "Key Issues in Developing School-linked, Integrated Services." *The Future of Children* 2, 1: 85-94.

Gardner, S. (1994). "Conclusion." In *The Politics of Linking Schools and Social Services*, edited by L.A. Adler and S. Gardner. Washington, D.C.: The Falmer Press.

Gore, A. (1993). *From Red Tape to Results: Creating a Government that Works Better and Costs Less: Report of the National*

Performance Review. Washington, D.C.: U.S. Government Printing Office.

Guthrie, G.P., and L.F. Guthrie. (September, 1991). "Streamlining Interagency Collaboration for Youth At Risk." *Educational Leadership* 49, 1: 17-22.

Heath, S.B., and M.W. McLaughlin. (1989). "Policies for Children with Multiple Needs." In *Conditions of Children in California* (pp. 303-319). Berkeley, Calif.: Policy Analysis for California Education (PACE). (ERIC Document Reproduction Service No. ED 316 933)

Herman, J.L., L.L. Morris, and C.T. Fitz-Gibbon. (1987). *Evaluator's Handbook*. Newbury Park, Calif.: Sage.

Hodgkinson, H.L. (1989). *The Same Client: The Demographics of Education and Service Delivery Systems*. Washington, D.C.: Institute for Educational Leadership, Center for Demographic Policy.

Kanter, R. (1992). *When Giants Learn to Dance*. New York: Simon & Schuster.

Kirst, M. (January 1992). "Financing School-Linked Services." In *University of Southern California Policy Brief*. Los Angeles: U.S. Center for Research in Education Finance (CHEF).

Kirst, M. (1993). "Financing School-Linked Services." *Education and Urban Society* 25, 2: 166-174.

Kirst, M., and M.W. McLaughlin. (1989). "Rethinking Children's Policy." In *National Society for the Study of Education (NSEE) Yearbook*. Chicago: University of Chicago Press.

Levy, J.E., and W. Shepardson. (1992). "Look at Current School-linked Service Efforts." *The Future of Children* 2, 1: 44-55.

Louis, K.S., and M.B. Miles. (1990). *Improving the Urban High School: What Works and Why*. New York: Teachers College Press.

McCart, L. (1993). *Changing Systems for Children and Families*. Washington, D.C.: National Governor's Association.

McLaughlin, M. W. (1990). "The Rand Change Agent Study Revisited: Macro Perspectives and Micro Realities." *Educational Researcher* 19, 9: 11-16.

Melaville, A.I., and M.J. Blank. (1991). *What it Takes: Structuring Interagency Partnerships to Connect Children and Families with Comprehensive Services*. Washington, D.C.: Education and Human Services Consortium.

Melaville, A.I., and M.J. Blank. (1993). *Together We Can: A Guide for Creating a Profamily System of Education and Human Services*. Washington, D.C.: U.S. Department of Education, U.S. Department of Health and Human Services.

REFERENCES

Mitchell, D., and L. Scott. (1994). "Professional and Institutional Perspectives on Interagency Collaboration." In *The Politics of Linking Schools and Social Services*, edited by L. Adler and S. Gardner. New York: Falmer Press.

New Beginnings Team. (1990). *New Beginnings: A Feasibility Study of Integrated Services for Children and Families*. (Final report and appendices). San Diego, Calif.: Office of the Deputy Superintendent, San Diego City Schools.

Olson, L. (November 2, 1994). "Learning Their Lessons." *Education Week*, 43-46.

Osborne, D., and T. Gaebler. (1993). *Reinventing Government: How the Entrepreneurial Spirit is Transforming the Public Sector*. New York: Penguin Books.

Payzant, T. (October 1992). "New Beginnings in San Diego: Developing a Strategy for Interagency Collaboration." *Phi Delta Kappan* 74, 2: 139 - 146.

Russo, C.J., and J.C. Lindle. (1994). "On the Cutting Edge: Family Resource/Youth Service Centers in Kentucky." In *The Politics of Linking Schools and Social Services*, edited by L.A. Adler and S. Gardner. Washington, D.C.: The Falmer Press.

Schorr, L.B. (1988). *Within Our Reach: Breaking the Cycle of Disadvantage*. New York: Anchor Press.

Senge, P. (1990). *The Fifth Discipline: The Art and Practice of the Learning Organization*. New York: Doubleday.

Smolowe, J. (February 1994). "...And Throw Away the Key." *Time*, 55-59.

U.S. Department of Housing and Urban Development. (1988). Partners in *Self-sufficiency Guidebook*. (ED 314 531). Washington, D.C.: Author.

Wagner, M., D. Shaver, L. Newman, M. Wechsler, F. Kelley, and S. Golan. (1994). *Implementing School-Linked Services: A Process Evaluation of the First Year of California's Healthy Start Initiative*. Menlo Park, Calif.: SRI International.